START LOVING YOUR
SMILE

DR. F. EDWARD MURDOCH

START LOVING YOUR
SMILE

THE INSIDER'S GUIDE TO
ORTHODONTIC CARE

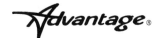

Published by Advantage, Charleston, South Carolina.
Member of Advantage Media Group.

ADVANTAGE is a registered trademark, and the Advantage colophon is a trademark of Advantage Media Group, Inc.

Printed in the United States of America.

10 9 8 7 6 5 4 3 2 1

ISBN: 978-1-64225-014-5
LCCN: 2019934686

Cover design by George Stevens
Layout design by Megan Elger

This publication is designed to provide accurate and authoritative information in regard to the subject matter covered. It is sold with the understanding that the publisher is not engaged in rendering legal, accounting, or other professional services. If legal advice or other expert assistance is required, the services of a competent professional person should be sought.

Advantage Media Group is proud to be a part of the Tree Neutral® program. Tree Neutral offsets the number of trees consumed in the production and printing of this book by taking proactive steps such as planting trees in direct proportion to the number of trees used to print books. To learn more about Tree Neutral, please visit www.treeneutral.com.

Advantage Media Group is a publisher of business, self-improvement, and professional development books. We help entrepreneurs, business leaders, and professionals share their Stories, Passion, and Knowledge to help others Learn & Grow. Do you have a manuscript or book idea that you would like us to consider for publishing? Please visit advantagefamily.com or call 1.866.775.1696.

TABLE OF CONTENTS

Foreword

From the Founder of Excellence in Orthodontics

MY NAME IS DR. DUSTIN BURLESON. I'm an orthodontist and the founder of Excellence in Orthodontics. My reasons for becoming an orthodontist and forming a national organization for exceptionally successful orthodontists leading the field in both clinical and patient care—instead of becoming a veterinarian or handsome movie actor or professor of poetry—are easily found at ExcellenceinOrthodontics.org, if you're curious. They might matter to you.

But this book is about *you*, the parent, and your son or daughter, not about me. It's about information you need to know to make intelligent, responsible decisions about your child's health, appearance, self-esteem, and social interactions … of a permanent, lifelong nature. Does your child really *need* braces? If so, when? If so, who should you trust to provide their orthodontic care? How will you know you're not being ripped off?

This book isn't *Fifty Shades of Gray*. It just can't be that exciting. But if you take the time to read this book, you'll know how to confidently and correctly make whatever decisions you need to make about your child's orthodontic care.

It's *not* 1982.

To start, we're no longer dealing with heavy, ugly, tight, painful metal braces—every visit to have them tightened was another round of torture; they were hard to put on, hard to keep on, painful to remove, and it was irritating having a list of foods and activities to avoid for a long period of time. If your child needs braces now, the experience won't be anything like it was when you were a kid. They won't even try hiding under the bed and have to be dragged kicking and screaming to the car.

Not only has *everything* about braces changed, but now all braces are created differently. So try to get that horrible, metal-mouth image out of your head. You're probably aware of invisible braces, maybe by a brand name: Invisalign. That's what prompts a lot of patients to call or email me in the first place. However, Invisalign is but one of a number of options to be considered to get to *the* best, customized, and personalized answer to your child's needs. You don't want to equate this to buying something over the counter: "Hey, give me Invisalign. How much?" It's more complicated than that. But it's a good representation of modern braces. They can be (nearly) invisible, pliable, safer, and even self-removable for hygiene or sports and easily put back in place. They're not painful and achieve more certain results in a shorter period of time.

When I was growing up, a lot of kids didn't get braces they really needed and their parents let them off the hook, either because they believed their child couldn't tolerate the pain or because the cost was just beyond the family's budget. Now that braces are virtually painless, what about the cost?

Today's far better braces cost *less* than the one-size-fits-all, metal-mouth braces of the '60s, '70s, and '80s. They cost as little as one Starbucks drink a day for a year, rarely more than twice that, and there are a number of different payment plans available if needed. So, that second hurdle is a lot lower than it was when our parents encountered it.

In other words, the first of my two introductory messages is: *relax*.

I've got your back. It's going to be okay—better than okay, easier than okay, and more convenient than okay. Orthodontic procedures *won't* hurt your child, and he or she will surprise you by not complaining it does. It's *not* going to hurt your bank account; you won't be reduced to a backyard stay-cation next summer and the summer after that. It's *not* going to be a maddening maelstrom of appointments of uncertain length, or hours in a waiting room: no emergencies from broken wires and loose braces.

More Than Just Braces

My second introductory message is: this is about more than just braces.

Orthodontic care for a child, preteen, or teen is more than just correcting crooked, crowded teeth with braces. That's like thinking diabetes only needs attention when feet have to be amputated, or getting tires checked might be a good idea after being stranded with a flat at night while it's pouring rain.

"Thank you for making our experience with braces pleasant and happy. As a busy working mom, I never knew it would be this easy and affordable."

—MARIA R.

Orthodontic checkups *by an orthodontist*[1], starting at age eight or nine, are a proper part of child rearing. In many cases, prevention is less troublesome and less costly. Even if you're late getting your son or daughter in, it's still possible they won't need braces and that other treatment options will do. But if they do need braces, the sooner you know of the options, the better.

This is also about more than just braces because it impacts psychological and emotional health, not just oral health. This is discussed later in the book.

Why It's Important

1. Straight teeth function better, are easier to clean, and are more likely to last a lifetime.

2. People with straight, well-aligned teeth can avoid gum disease, which has very serious health ramifications.

3. Properly aligned jaws reduce the risk of temporomandibular joint disorders (TMJ), which can ruin sleep or cause chronic headaches or migraines.

4. Both kids and adults with great smiles feel better about themselves, and that can greatly increase their confidence.

Some parents put off orthodontic treatment, but these irregularities and problems do *not* heal themselves. *This isn't acne; they don't grow out of it.* The problems only grow worse and harder to resolve with age.

---

1   All orthodontists are dentists, but dentists are *not* the same as or suitable substitutes for orthodontists. Read on to find out more.

Don't Ask Them to Hide Their Smile

Never smiling isn't easy in an age of selfies and social media. Children can become self-conscious—painfully self-conscious—and embarrassed. "No thanks, Mom, I'd rather just stay home."

Teen suicide has skyrocketed since social media shaming and bullying rose to ugly prominence. Teen depression affects everything from getting the good grades needed to get into a good college to first dates, first loves, and enjoying (or hating) their childhood and teen years. But it doesn't stop there. Uncorrected, bad smiles go with them to college and into their career.

This isn't just cosmetic either. It is medical and can be a serious detriment to their health.

So, read on. Be informed. Be able to ask smart questions and do the right thing. I guarantee you'll be much better able to correctly and confidently make good choices for your family through this book.

Dr. Dustin S. Burleson, DDS

Founder, Excellence in Orthodontics

Clinical Professor, The University of Missouri Kansas City School of Dentistry, Department of Graduate Orthodontics & Dentofacial Orthopedics

Adjunct Professor, The Children's Mercy Hospital, Kansas City, Missouri, Department of Cleft & Craniofacial Orthodontics

Director, The Rheam Foundation for Cleft & Craniofacial Orthodontics

Introduction

A Little About Me and the Importance of Family....

I WAS BORN AND RAISED in Fredericton, New Brunswick. Fredericton is a beautiful city with amazing people who I was fortunate to grow up with. I am proud to count my family members among those people—our families are the most important people in our lives and inspire us to do what we do.

My father was a dentist, and in his early years in practice, people would be lined up at the door to have their problem teeth pulled. The amount of dental disease in the community bothered my father so much that he felt we needed more prevention and proactivity in our community. He recruited and brought the first dental hygienist to town to teach his patients about dental health and prevention of dental disease.

My mother was also in healthcare as a nurse and, later in life, she became the executive director of the local lung association. This was at a time when most people smoked in our community, and there was little education and awareness about the long-term effects. My mom was proactive in setting up smoking cessation classes and spreading awareness of preventing lung disease. In addition, she was an innovator introducing "lung runs" into the community and summer activity camps set up for kids that struggled growing up with asthma.

As her son, I was recruited, along with my siblings, to participate as camp leaders. Through that experience, I learned a lot about children struggling with health concerns.

I grew up with two older sisters and a younger brother. Having experienced life in a small community and having two parents as healthcare providers, it was inevitable that we all ended up choosing an education in healthcare.

The older of my two sisters lives in Michigan and is also a dentist, but she has chosen to go to a higher-level by educating dentists. She is now the associate dean at the University of Michigan School of Dentistry. She has a passion for the profession and educating the future generations of dentists and hygienists. And she was really instrumental in setting the bar high for me and my siblings. I couldn't be prouder of her accomplishments.

The younger of the two sisters chose to become a pharmacist and met her husband while in pharmacy school. She is the kindest, caring person you could ever meet and I am confident she makes a difference every day in her patients' lives, including those in nursing homes.

My brother and I both have a passion for sports. We're one year apart, and he was a great friend and teammate to me. He chose medical school instead of dentistry, but excelled while there and went on to specialize as an anesthesiologist.

When I started to write this book, it made me reflect on why I do what I do; I thought of my family, and it became clear. Growing up, we would always sit around the dinner table and talk about how to make a difference in our communities. From these mealtime discussions, healthcare was baked into all of us. In particular, preventive care before patients suffered from other health complications just made sense to all of us.

I was destined to follow my dad and older sister, so I entered dental school, where I developed a keen interest in growth and development as well as treating a patient's whole smile through preventive and corrective means. It became apparent to me that the most impact I could have on a patient's health and well-being was through orthodontics. It became my passion.

Once I completed dental school at Dalhousie University in Halifax, Nova Scotia, I headed out west to discover more of Canada and set up to practice in Vancouver. I admit, the outdoor life, climate, and recreation—especially skiing—was a draw, along with the open mindset of the people who live on the West Coast.

I worked in the Vancouver area as a general dentist at multiple practices for five years, and also taught at the University of British Columbia in the paediatric dentistry department. I pursued orthodontic training at the general dentist level but discovered how much more complex the specialty was and how limited my skills would be. I knew that, to get proper training, I would need to go back to school so I could treat my patients to the level they deserve!

I applied and got accepted at a number of orthodontic programs, but I chose Eastman Dental Centre at the University of Rochester in New York because of its reputation and the man who led the program for decades, Dr. Daniel Subtelny. Dr. Subtelny, and the orthodontists he attracted to teach in the program, lead the field in innovative approaches to the most complex problems, including cleft palate treatments, surgical treatments, lingual orthodontic techniques—and especially growth, development, and preventive approaches.

He was someone who had a great influence on me and I respect him very much. His teaching method was to make us think deeply about problems at hand as well as think outside the box for solutions.

During this time in the United States, my wife and I had two children and met people in the program from all over the world. We made some really good friends and were exposed to different cultures and different ways of thinking. We also layered a New York accent on top of our maritime accent, which was quite an interesting combination and kept people guessing at where we were from.

Once finishing school in New York, we decided to head back to the west coast of Canada and put down roots on Vancouver Island. We were drawn to the ocean and all the island has to offer. What a great place to raise our family!

I've been in orthodontics since 1996. It is truly an amazing profession and it's unbelievable how much it's changed over the years. It has never been easier and less time consuming for patients to get the smile transformation that orthodontics can create.

Apart from just doing orthodontics, I've spent a lot of time working as a team with other dentists and surgeons to reconstruct patients' smiles. I belong to and mentor a couple of dental study groups, including one famous in dentistry called "Spear Education," which is a truly amazing program and group of people based in Scottsdale, Arizona.

What I learned from a lot of these patients is that although they are grateful when they finish their treatment, they've ultimately had to invest a lot of time and money to rehabilitate their mouth and smile. When I look at them and talk about their care, they often say they wished they had known about the problems and dealt with them earlier in life as a teenager so they could have prevented a lot of issues from happening. I really feel that dental awareness and education is so important and that is why I've written this book. Preventive dentistry is really not talked about as much as it should be. I see it daily in my practice and I want to help people be aware of these problems so they can prevent them.

You have one smile and one set of teeth for your whole life. They are not just for eating and looks but serve an important part of our social interaction and our overall health; they are involved in almost everything in life—not only the basics of eating, speaking, and breathing, but also our confidence, first impressions, first kisses, and most importantly, overall body health, including cardiovascular health.

If we can get families and the kids in those families in for an orthodontic checkup when they are young and developing—and help them understand dental health and taking care of their teeth—then we can save them from a lot of problems down the road as well as increase their confidence and success that comes from that.

We have developed a program to train our team members as advocates and coaches for our patients and their smiles. Their primary directive and mission is to be advocates for people's oral health and coach them along the way. Through education growth and an emphasis on prevention, we hope to change dentistry through this more modern approach.

People, especially teens, need us to explain why we are doing what we do. Kids today want to understand things and engage through images and videos, not just by being told what to do and how to do it. We find that by using the innovative tools available to us now, we can engage people early on in life, and in turn, they will value what they have and what can be created so that they may have the best smile and take care of it for life.

When my children were young, I decided to take up surfing, mostly at the urging of my kids when we visited Tofino. Let me tell you—it is not an easy sport. But I love the challenge! I was at a lecture listening to an orthodontist from Hawaii who compared orthodontics with surfing and this, of course, piqued my interest. He showed a huge wave with many people on it. One guy was ripping across the face of the wave, and many other people were on the other side of the wave that were unable to catch it. They didn't have the knowledge or confidence to go for it. That guy was Laird Hamilton, a professional surfer, and on closer inspection, we saw that many of them had the same board as him, yet he was the only one who had spent the time and made the effort to be his very best so he could tackle it. It was a bit unfair since it was his specialty and full-time job. The rest of the surf crew were likely weekend warriors and hobbyists. So, of course, he was the only one who could navigate all it took to catch and surf the wave. I found that a great analogy for most things in my life—however, my full-time job is orthodontics. Surfing—not so much, I'm just one of the weekend warriors!

However, like the weekend warriors wanting to catch the wave in the picture, many dentists have access to the tools like braces and Invisalign (like the surfers had access to professional surfboards), but not many people have dedicated the time and effort needed to master the skills to be the best they can be at this one special thing. It's just "another thing they can do."

I enjoy learning so much and embrace anything that is innovative, especially the changes in our profession with technology. That is why I am so excited with how much has been brought into our industry and how it is changing for the better. The products are better—we are looking at things in 3-D instead of 2-D and we use digital tools and treatment planning to help us get to the end point in the most direct way possible. For the patient, this means less discomfort, which equates to less time in the chair. This flows into less time missing school or work, less time to get to the finish line, and less time not being able to eat what they want! It's all good!

I hope this book will answer any questions you may have about orthodontics. It truly is amazing the difference we can make in people's lives. This is what I love about preventive healthcare in general, and my specialty in particular!

We often have a young girl or boy come into our office very shy and embarrassed about their teeth, and their transformation is wonderful—to see them come out of their shell and become more self-confident. There is no better time than in these formative years. And with our adult patients that have wanted to have treatment since they were teens, there is no better time than now.

Chapter One

Why Is My Child's Smile So Important?

IF YOU ARE WEIGHING the yes/no and now/later decisions of orthodontic care or braces, you'll be trying to decide just how important or unimportant it really is.

Some parents feel "looks aren't everything." Some think their kid should just be tough-minded about this and not overly sensitive. Some may not have had orthodontic care when they were children and think, *Hey, I turned out just fine. I have a great spouse, a good career, friends—so what's the big deal?*

This isn't *just* a cosmetic issue. Misaligned, crooked teeth could cause *significant* medical problems.

Poorly aligned teeth can produce chronic headaches and migraines, contribute to digestive problems because of the inability to properly chew foods, and make getting a decent night's sleep impossible. Perhaps the most dangerous of all: it can foster gum disease. Gum disease has absolute links to diabetes, heart disease, strokes and dementia, as well as, of course, the loss of natural teeth altogether. Orthodontic corrections later in adult life can be more difficult and involved due to wear on the teeth over time.

Uncorrected mouth problems and misaligned teeth make for strangely stretched gums inevitably destined to separate from teeth. This could allow "pockets" for infections and periodontal disease to arise and turn into *very* difficult, painful, and costly problems late in life.

In the teenage years, failure to spend money on orthodontic treatment can easily cost ten times that amount in full mouth restoration case at age forty or fifty, or embarrassing, health-compromising removal of all teeth and use of dentures at age sixty.

Gum disease is serious business. It worsens the risks of and heightens dangers from diabetes, heart disease, strokes, and dementia. Ignoring preteen or teen teeth misalignment may virtually guarantee adult medical problems. If there is a genetic history of any of these medical problems I just named, you only worsen the odds of your son or daughter suffering from them by ignoring or postponing needed orthodontic treatment.

Aside from impacting health, a poorly aligned smile can significantly impact your child's comfort. Headaches, toothaches, sinus problems, dry mouth, snoring, drooling, bad breath, and insomnia are all symptoms of a smile that isn't straight, jaws that aren't aligned, or teeth that are too close together or not quite close enough. Oftentimes, however, the mouth is the last place we check for signs of discomfort, loss of sleep, or even a simple headache.

If your child's pediatrician can't figure out why they're not sleeping well or experiencing headaches or even insomnia for which there seems to be no cause, a simple thirty-minute exam at your local orthodontist could provide a clear solution in no time!

Here is what I'm told by an awful lot of parents:

> "I had wonderful parents, *but* I sure wish they had found a way to afford the braces I needed and gotten me the care I needed when I was a kid, so I didn't grow up to have this bad smile my whole life."

And what I hear from almost every adult patient getting orthodontic treatment and braces is:

> "I had wonderful parents, *but* I sure wish they had found a way to afford the braces I needed and gotten me the care I needed when I was a kid, so I didn't grow up to have this bad smile my whole life *and have all these problems now.*"

Is this how you want your daughter or son talking about you ten, twenty, or thirty years from now? Is this how you want them remembering their childhood?

If that sounds pretty damned pushy, I admit: it is. I kept it in the book for the very simple reason that this is *truly* what I have heard so much over the years, and I am sincere about letting you reflect on it. All parents want to do the right thing. They don't want to let their children down in any way, and I'm sure you don't either.

Parents will do anything they can to afford paying for their kids' college, trying their best to guide the decision, trekking around the country on campus visits, worrying over campus culture, or taking on *serious* debt. Every parent understands what many kids can't—that it's not about the few years of college but rather the forty or fifty years afterward.

I assure you, this is the same. It's not about the bad, humiliating smile and bad bite transformed now, for high school. It's about the many, many years to come. They really can't appreciate that now, but *you* can.

No parent wants their child to suffer, either from teeth that actually hurt, headaches you can't explain, insomnia that affects their daily life, or insecurity your child may be feeling because of a crooked or oversized smile. The fact is, your child's formative years are actually the most sensitive for his or her teeth. Now is the time to pay close attention to your child's smile, behavior, peer relationships, and confidence level.

If any or all are lacking, a qualified orthodontist may help give you and your child the peace of mind you both crave.

The Top Five Reasons People Avoid Seeing the Orthodontist

1. **Patients are afraid it's going to hurt.** Pain is the number-one reason most people avoid going to the orthodontist. However, modern technology—and choosing the right orthodontist—can ensure that your child enjoys a pain-free orthodontic experience.

2. **Patients are afraid it's going to cost too much.** Not only are most orthodontic procedures more affordable than ever, but insurance, payment plans, and a variety of other financing options make this all but a moot point for most of my patients. Remember, orthodontists aren't in this to get rich, they're here to make sure your child's teeth, smile, and jaw are

aligned to make his or her life better—period! We're not going to let something like price get in the way of creating a better, safer, healthier smile for your child.

3. **Patients are afraid it's going to take too long / they're going to miss too much school or work.** Regardless of the type of orthodontic procedure your child needs, time is of the essence. Modern technology and ease of access allows us to work around your child's school schedule with minimal absences. After initial visits, and barring the actual procedure itself, most visits and/or adjustments are routine and can take anywhere from fifteen to forty-five minutes and can be scheduled conveniently.

4. **Patients do not see the need to take action.** Eroding, crooked, or unaligned smiles can take time to happen, but the time to act is now. Orthodontic irregularities don't just heal on their own or disappear if you ignore them. Your child's smile and overall dental health are too important to ignore out of questions of pain, convenience, or even price.

5. **Patients have been treated in the past with an attitude of indifference.** Let's face it, not all doctors are created equal. Every profession has its "bad apples," and to say dentistry is the exception would be to write fiction instead of fact. There is no room for indifference when it comes to your child's healthcare. Find an orthodontic specialist that offers not only state of the art technology for your child, but state of the art service as well. Orthodontic special-

ists know what it's like to sit in the chair, and should provide every opportunity for patients, especially our younger patients, to feel comfortable, safe, and secure in our care.

Chapter Two

Why Do Kids Need Braces?

ARE BRACES SOMETHING CREATED by orthodontists to make money, like Disney and their extra-charge FastPass? Was it a conspiracy from the very start?

Then and now, there may be some overprescribing and premature prescribing by some doctors. There are bad apples in every orchard. And you know the adage: if all he's got is a hammer, everything (and everybody) looks like a nail.

But there is a very legitimate, clinically documented, and 90 percent of the time, clearly visible reason why some kids, as young as eight, *need* orthodontic treatment and care: malocclusion.

Malocclusion is mostly genetic, so if your daughter or son has it, blame their grandparents. It's a fancy-pants term for all things related to misaligned teeth—teeth growing angled, crooked, and into a too-crowded space. It can be a single tooth, a few teeth, or the whole mouth. There can be other causes too, like early, premature loss of primary teeth, chronic thumb-sucking, or even an accident that seemed to leave no lasting effect at its moment in time.

If your child is suffering from any, several, or all of the following early indicators of malocclusion, consider having them addressed by an orthodontic specialist sooner rather than later:

- **Crossbites**: A crossbite occurs when the jaw deviates to one side with an improper fit of the upper and lower teeth from left to right or front to back. Crossbites can lead to worn and chipped teeth, jaw pain, and asymmetric growth of the jaws. Left untreated, the crossbite may require more extensive treatment later in life.

- **Thumb-sucking**: Thumb-sucking habits beginning at the age of seven or older should be corrected immediately in order to prevent severe jaw and tooth alignment problems.

- **Miscellaneous concerns**: There are several associated issues you should also be looking for as soon as your child turns seven in order to intervene early, including the following:

  □ permanent teeth that are growing into the wrong spots

  □ severely protruded front teeth at risk for injury

  □ severe crowding with permanent teeth erupting into poor-quality gum tissue

With any of these situations, we can discuss the pros and cons of early intervention and treatment versus waiting until all the permanent teeth are in for orthodontic correction. If you are anxious about the appearance of your child's teeth or your child is self-conscious about his or her appearance, early treatment might be the best choice. Not only are most orthodontic problems more difficult to correct later, but self-image and personality inhibition can be hard for a person to leave behind. However, if your child is extremely resistant to braces or is not mature enough to be trusted to care for them, delay may be the better choice. In that case, regularly scheduled orthodontic checkups will be necessary.

Having malocclusion does *not* guarantee a child will need orthodontic therapy. Frankly, this is what worries me about nonspecialists like family dentists substituting themselves for orthodontists, and parents letting it happen. They may easily miss an early diagnosis of malocclusion, when it could have been treated without braces. Or they may leap to braces as the only way to treat all malocclusion. Either way, you and your child lose.

The first question, then, is: does your child have or show all the signs they are going to have malocclusion? Second, if so, what—of numerous options—should be done about it? Third, when?

To have all these questions answered early, the first full orthodontic exam should occur early in a child's life. I recommend seven or eight, no later than nine, especially if there is family history of malocclusion. With early and periodic exams by an orthodontic specialist, you may avoid their need for orthodontic therapy and/or you may prevent years of suffering and embarrassment related to their teeth and smile.

Waiting will have very serious consequences, often requiring more treatment and higher costs later in life. What most parents fail to realize is that these treatment problems are urgent and should be treated as such. If that ship has sailed, the next best time for a full orthodontic exam is tomorrow at three o'clock.

If your child does need orthodontic therapy—now or at some predictable future time—the outcome of the exam can lead to *sensible* decisions. If not now, treatment to prevent the need can begin, and also, you can begin saving money for orthodontics or other procedures if necessary later on in your child's life. There is no tooth fairy coming to leave a few thousand dollars underneath their pillow or yours. But if the need must be met three years from now, skipping one Starbucks run a week for those three years can make a hefty dent in the bill to come. How to fund orthodontic treatment is discussed later in the book.

Let me be emphatically clear. I am *not* in the business of putting any child through orthodontic therapy if they don't need it. My office is *not* a braces store. I'm in the business of helping kids and families get the right appliance if any is needed, get the right braces if any are needed, and have as perfect a smile and as few oral health problems as possible. I make sure my patients are informed—that's why I wrote this book. In my office, you're never told what to do. You're provided with real information, no medical jargon, plain English, "reasons why," and options. You probably know the term "God complex," referring to a person who acts like he's God—imperious, brusque, and deliberately intimidating to squash questions. You will *not* get that kind of treatment here, from me or anyone on my team.

Kids do need orthodontic therapy, but not all kids and certainly not the same appliances for all. Some kids are better served by other limited interceptive treatments instead of or before comprehensive orthodontic therapy. We will collaborate, you and I, to figure out what is or isn't needed and what options are best if there is a need for your child.

Chapter Three

Why Not Just a Dentist?
Why an Orthodontist?

YOU UNDOUBTEDLY ALREADY have a dentist.

Gee, isn't seeing an orthodontist going to cost a lot more?

I'm busy. More appointments?

Do I really need to get orthodontic checkups for my kids?

Don't worry, these are all reasonable questions! It is true that, today, quite a few dentists dance over into our territory, and although they're *not* permitted to claim they're the same as orthodontists or provide orthodontic treatment (beware of any who do), they're able to do things like provide Invisalign and braces. This can be confusing. Here are the facts.

All orthodontists are dentists and we all graduate from the same dental schools. True enough. But that's where it stops for dentists. Orthodontists go to school for an additional two to three years to become credentialed specialists at diagnosing and providing the best treatment for conditions like:

- difficulties chewing or biting
- constant biting into the cheek, gums, or roof of the mouth
- teeth that meet abnormally or don't meet at all
- teeth grinding or clenching
- crowded, misplaced, or blocked out teeth
- early or late loss of teeth
- teeth grown in badly
- teeth that protrude
- embarrassing personal appearance due to teeth
- facial imbalances
- teeth or jaw misalignment, TMJ
- chronic headaches and migraine
- poor sleep
- speech difficulties (that may never be outgrown or may develop later)

These are *not* dental care issues. They are orthodontic issues. The appliances used in orthodontics are tools, and their success rate is highly dependant on the skill, training, and experience of the operator.

You could go to a buddy and ask him to build you a garage because he owns a hammer and nails, but what kind of result do you expect? However, if this same friend owned a home renovation company or is a building contractor, you'd expect far superior results, wouldn't you?

For *some* things, a generalist or jack-of-all-trades will do. For other things, you know it's smart to seek out the best specialist you can afford. For example, if, come tax time, you have simple, ordinary deductions, getting your taxes prepared for the cheapest fee at the seasonal H&R Block office that opens up in your neighborhood shopping center is probably fine. But if you have more complications with investment income from real estate, depreciation on real estate, own stocks, and you raise iguanas as a money hobby, you're going to get yourself a really good accountant, probably a CPA. If you need the simplest will, leaving everything first to spouse or second to daughter may be okay. But if you are of some means and have several children and maybe also grandchildren as well as charities, you're going to need to see an *estate planning* attorney, not just any attorney—though they all went to the same law schools—but *a specialist in estate planning.*

This is no different.

There are a few things to keep in mind when differentiating between a general dentist and an orthodontic specialist.

First, general dentists, or jacks-of-all-trades, tend to work with one-size-fits-all, off-the-rack, standardized solutions. They likely do only a few treatments per year. They may be limited to doing only what the computer software dictates that they do when planning a case, without bringing experience, expertise, and expert judgment to bear. They're often working with products from only one provider, without being able to select from a full range of options that would work best for you. Orthodontic specialists, instead, do hundreds of cases each year and use this experience and their full arsenal of tools to individually and carefully diagnose needs and provide personalized solutions.

Second, generalists and their use of inexpertly applied, standardized solutions tend to be cheaper than the fees of a specialist, but that also places economic pressure on them to do the treatment as quickly and simply as possible, because they've "cut it thin."

In this case, it's worth remembering that the treatment provided has permanent, lifelong, and life-impacting consequences. This concerns your health, future dental or jaw alignment or misalignment issues affecting quality of sleep (which can affect weight, even onset and management of type 2 diabetes and heart disease), as well as self-esteem and social and career success.

General Dentist. A general dentist gives routine checkups, preventive measures, cleans teeth, and fixes cavities. They may not start seeing children until they are seven to ten years old.

Pediatric Dentist. A pediatric dentist has two to three years of specialized education beyond dental school. They specialize in providing dental care to children and adolescents, offering checkups, preventive measures, cleanings, and cavities.

Orthodontist. An orthodontist has two to three years of specialized education *beyond* dental school and is an expert at straightening teeth and aligning the jaws. They assess patients and determine the best treatment routes and procedures that need to be taken.

If you can, you want to choose an orthodontist for orthodontic care.

You may ask, *how do I know my doctor is an orthodontist?* It's a good question and a critical one to ask as you seek additional treatment for your child's dental issues.

Only orthodontists can belong to the American Association of Orthodontists (AAO). If you're looking for a local orthodontist, go online and visit **www.braces.org** to find a specialist in your area. This website features not only a searchable database of orthodontists but educational tips, answers and resources to help you on your quest for your child's healthiest smile!

Alternatively, you can ask your doctor if he or she has completed a two- to three-year residency in orthodontics and check with your provincial board to follow up on their reply. Dentists and orthodontists in most provinces will be registered differently with the dental board.

Do your homework; be a "dental detective" while on the hunt for such vital information. Look for the words "dental specialist in orthodontics," or ask your general dentist for a referral to a specialist. In urban and suburban areas, it will take minimal effort to find a specialist. In more remote, rural locations, your search might take you to another city or town. Don't be afraid to ask your dentist if an orthodontist travels to your town every month to see patients. There's a chance an orthodontist from a larger city comes to your town and works out of another dental office once or twice per month. Looking around can save valuable driving time and money.

One note: there is no disrespect between orthodontists and dentists. As a matter of fact, many orthodontic patients are referred by their dentists. These are great, capable, and caring professionals who know where their expertise begins and ends, and who do not let ego or income opportunity step in front of what they know is best for their patients. Just as the family doctor refers his patients with possible or significant heart disease issues to a cardiologist, and if need be, the cardiologist refers to a surgeon, the best dentists refer patients with orthodontic needs to orthodontists. Orthodontists are required to take two to three years of university education beyond dental school and additional continuing clinical education every year. They must also invest in state-of-the-art technology for their offices (not found in dental offices)—*all for a good reason.*

Even though we orthodontists have the education and training to perform general dentist procedures, we don't. We specialize.

Chapter Four

Choose the Right Orthodontist

What are some good clues to selecting a great orthodontist?

I've got two: their practice is busy.

When you see a really, really busy practice, there are probably a whole lot of patient referrals, and neither kids nor parents enthusiastically refer if they feel they were lied to or treated badly, put in pain, or wound up with results nothing like the digital future-photo they were shown. And they probably wouldn't come to that practice if they had to keep coming back to "fix a few things," or were overcharged. Parents tell parents about great orthodontic practices because we earned their trust and because their kids keep thanking them.

This is a business, a business built on ethics and earned trust. And you do *not* just need a doctor to install orthodontic appliances; you need a trustworthy advisor.

The other clue: a great orthodontist is *not* cheap.

Our fees are calculated to allow for "Cadillac + Care" in every respect, to put no downward financial pressure on how we care for patients and parents, and to *never* cut corners or take shortcuts. We *never* use any material that is "probably good enough."

If I were you, I'd worry if I could find an orthodontist that is a lot cheaper. If you do find one, know this: behind closed doors they're probably asking, "Can we do this cheaper?" Is *that* the question you want discussed back there, at every step of your child's treatment?

There's a science and an art to this. Me and my staff are all highly trained to produce state-of-the-art outcomes, nothing less. The doctor makes a difference. That's why I tell everybody to get a highly successful orthodontist.

The Top Ten Things You Should Know *Before* Choosing Your Orthodontist

This is something you want to be sure about. I've just suggested one big consideration: a very successful practice. Here are ten more.

1. Are they a specialist?

Orthodontists are specially trained and have extensive experience transforming smiles. All orthodontists are dentists, but only 6 percent of dentists are orthodontists. An additional two to three years of specialized education qualifies orthodontists to expertly identify, diagnose, and treat a broad spectrum of dental irregularities such as early or late loss of teeth, improper jaw alignment or fit, speech difficulty, impacted teeth, grinding or clenching of teeth, and facial imbalance. Orthodontists look at more than just the "straightness" of the teeth. They consider the whole health of the head and neck, drawing on expertise developed over many years of experience treating similar cases, ensuring your treatment plan will be custom tailored to meet your unique needs and give you the results you deserve.

2. Do they treat adults as well as children?

Orthodontics is not just for kids! While we do believe that an ounce of prevention is worth a pound of cure, and that seeing and monitoring children from a young age can prevent or reduce the severity of many dental problems developing as they get older, we also firmly believe that it is never too late for straight teeth and a healthy bite. We often hear our adults comment about how they wanted, or should have had, braces when they were younger but never did. We pride ourselves on being able to make straight teeth a reality for our adult patients. There has never been a better time for orthodontic treatment. A healthy and attractive smile, and a perfect bite is important not only to a person's physical and dental health, but also to their confidence and the way they feel about themselves.

3. Do they provide the first visit free of charge?

Most orthodontists offer free examinations for new patients so you and your family can get expert advice about needs, options, and timing before making this important investment. Your first exam and consultation is a great time to make sure your questions are being answered, concerns are addressed, and you are being fully educated about all your treatment options.

We provide a complimentary examination and orthodontic consultation with images. During your first exam and consultation, we will be sure to answer any questions, address any concerns, and educate you about all your treatment options.

4. Do they offer a guarantee?

No matter which orthodontist you choose, ultimately, you are not making a small investment. That being said, wouldn't you want to ensure your orthodontist is going to stand behind their treatment?

Of course! At Ocean's Edge Orthodontics, we offer you a 100 percent satisfaction guarantee. If your satisfaction is less than 100 percent at any time, we simply ask you to inform us so that we can correct it. Our team will strive to make sure you are as relaxed and comfortable as possible throughout your orthodontic treatment.

5. Are they using the latest technology and treatment options available?

Orthodontics today differs a great deal from years past due to significant advances in technology. Computer-designed clear aligners (Invisalign), braces, and wires dramatically increase the precision with which teeth are moved. Clear braces offer a cosmetically pleasing alternative to regular braces, while Invisalign offers patients an entirely brace-free option. Did you know that Invisalign also has a special treatment system just for teens and children?

At Ocean's Edge Orthodontics, we guarantee that we can find the treatment option that will fit your lifestyle. In fact, I believe in staying current with the latest techniques, and offer 3-D imaging (including iCAT technology, iTero scanners, and treatment accelerating devices), and participating in international mastermind groups with some of the greatest orthodontic minds in North America. Ultimately, you get the most up-to-date treatment available when you choose Ocean's Edge Orthodontics.

6. Does their quoted fee include retainers?

Each orthodontic office has its own independently-considered fees reflecting the value of the treatment packages being offered. All orthodontists should offer you a contract that clearly spells out the treatment package for you or your child's treatment before it begins so you know exactly what it is you are paying for.

Retainers are a big part of your treatment. After you have worked so hard to achieve a beautiful smile, you want to keep it! Because of this, we provide extra retainers and 3-D printed models of your teeth so you have the tools to ensure your smile stays perfect forever!

7. Do they offer emergency appointments?

When researching an orthodontist in your area, be sure to ask whether his or her orthodontist office offers emergency/repair appointments and after-hours coverage. Your orthodontist should understand that emergencies and breakages do happen and be fully prepared in the event they do occur. Your orthodontist should explain to you the emergency procedure and steps to take to keep you comfortable throughout the process.

At Ocean's Edge Orthodontics, our Smile Coaches will give you simple dietary guidelines, plus care and usage coaching at every appointment to help you avoid extra visits due to repairs. We also understand that life happens so we have time built into our daily schedule and an after-hours care line to assist you when the need arises.

8. Do they make you feel special and comfortable?

Regardless if you are reading this book for your own treatment or for your child's treatment, when you meet with your orthodontist, you should feel comfortable and confident in your team.

We commit to making you feel part of our family and go above and beyond to ensure you have the best possible experience each time you visit. Our top priority is you.

9. Can they reduce your treatment time?

When it comes to orthodontics, patients often worry about the length of treatment. How long will you have to wear braces for? How long will you have to take care of them and avoid the foods you love? How much school or work will you have to miss due to appointments? These concerns and others may make you hesitant to go forward with the treatment you and your loved ones need.

At Ocean's Edge Orthodontics, we have invested in advanced tools and technology which allows us to help make your treatment progress as smoothly, as efficiently, and as quickly as possible, reducing the number of visits to our office and time away from work or school. For your convenience, we offer before and after school, evening, and occasional Saturday appointments to get you to "Smile Sooner"!

10. Do they offer flexible payment plans?

Once you are comfortable and you know which orthodontist you want to treat you or your child, the next questions are typically "how much is this going to cost?" and "how am I going to pay for this?"

At Ocean's Edge Orthodontics, you have lots of options! We will help you understand your payment options and will work with you to find a payment plan that will fit your budget and needs. We offer super-flexible, interest-free payment plans. If you have dental insurance, we will work with you to help you understand and maximize your benefits. Orthodontics is a significant investment and we want to make it as easy for you as we can.

11. (BONUS) Do they support the community?

We take pride in giving back to the communities that we live and work in. We support and donate to youth sports, the local school programs, and we provide low-cost treatment and braces to patients who cannot afford the full cost of treatment and have significant needs through the a program called "Smiles Change Lives" (we are the first provider in BC to participate in this fantastic program). Every child deserves a beautiful smile!

How to Know What Questions to Ask

I've really thought through the questions most parents and patients have—not just the ones they ask, but the ones they don't. This book attempts to cover them all, but again, this is a *personal* matter. The best questions to ask are the ones that matter most to you and your child.

I hope not, but you may be in a position that absolutely requires you to get the minimum essential treatment for the lowest cost. If so, your most important questions are going to be about those kinds of options and about price, and nothing else.

If, however, you are able to make your decision about who you should trust with your child's oral health and smile by many factors, we've included a "What Is Most Important to You?" quiz from Excellence In Orthodontics on the following pages. As you'll see, there are fourteen different items to consider and rank in importance to you. Any can become the questions you ask me and my team or any other orthodontist.

Incidentally, Excellence In Orthodontics is a national organization for exceptionally successful orthodontists leading the field in both clinical and patient care and patient/parent (client) service excellence. We all subscribe to a pledge of very high standards and hold each other accountable. You can learn more at ExcellenceInOrthdontics.org.

If you have a specific question not answered anywhere in this book, or have a personal and confidential question, you can—with complete assurance of privacy and courtesy—email StartLovingYourSmile@oeosmiles.com or call Dr. Edward Murdoch at 844-240-6688.

There is also a FAQ section at the back of this book.

Of course, a perfect opportunity to get questions answered— yours and your son's or daughter's—is at your exam appointment.

What Is Most Important to You?

Directions: For each **Key Item** below, rank its importance to you from 1 to 5. Then check off whether each type of provider provides that item. When you're done with all 14 Key Items, add up your rankings and review what your final score means about choosing an orthodontist.

	Key Items to Consider in Selecting Your Orthodontist	Rank How Important Each Item Is to You in Selecting Your Orthodontist 1 – Not Important, 5 – Very Important	Ocean's Edge Orthodontics	Other Provider	Other Provider
			Check Off If Provided		
1	Orthodontist and staff committed to expert, thorough diagnosis, and prescription of the best treatment plan customized for my son or daughter	1 2 3 4 5	✓		
2	Avoiding extractions (if possible)	1 2 3 4 5	✓		
3	Avoiding having to wear headgear with braces (if possible)	1 2 3 4 5	✓		
4	Avoiding "metal-mouth" braces (if possible) or utilizing the new type of "invisible" braces	1 2 3 4 5	✓		
5	Having a healthy, pleasing smile that will last a lifetime and protect optimum dental health (not just having straightened teeth)	1 2 3 4 5	✓		
6	Pain-free treatment	1 2 3 4 5	✓		
7	Orthodontist utilizes the most modern, advanced, and proven technology, including computer-aided design and fitting	1 2 3 4 5	✓		
8	Orthodontists and team actively involved in continuing clinical education	1 2 3 4 5	✓		
9	Reducing treatment time to a minimum without compromising results (including total length of treatment term and number of office visits)	1 2 3 4 5	✓		
10	Availability of after-school or after-work appointment options	1 2 3 4 5	✓		
11	Treatment coordinator is knowledgeable about insurance coverage and is able to offer flexible payment plans	1 2 3 4 5	✓		

12	Getting the best overall value factoring in thorough diagnosis, customized care, and concern with lifetime health and well-being—not just the cheapest fee	1	2	3	4	5	✔		
13	Lifetime guarantee	1	2	3	4	5	✔		
14	Orthodontist and team committed to excellence in orthodontics and customer service for both patients and parents	1	2	3	4	5	✔		

Total of Your Rankings

What Your Score Means

50-70 There is no doubt. Ocean's Edge Orthodontics is the right choice for you and your family! It is clear that you place a high value on a comprehensive, "best" approach.

43-49 You are probably also going to be happiest with Ocean's Edge Orthodontics, rather than any other alternative. But this score suggests you aren't completely sure and have some unanswered questions or concerns. Your doctor and the practice's treatment coordinator want no lingering uncertainties on your part, and want to address any and every question. Don't keep anything to yourself. Please ask.

42 or less Frankly, you may not value the advanced, sophisticated level of clinical care and customer service provided at Ocean's Edge Orthodontics. Cost may be much more important to you than other factors, or very basic service may be all you feel you need. It's perfectly okay. If you choose to shop around, be sure to use this checklist in evaluating other options. Remember, you do want everything right the first time, and you want error-free orthodontics at a minimum.

Chapter Five

What Can I Expect at the Initial Consultation and Exam?

MANY QUESTIONS SURROUND YOUR first visit to a new orthodontist, not the least of which is the subject of this particular chapter: *what will happen at the initial consultation?*

To answer this very common question, and perhaps several others you might not even realize you need answering yet, let me walk you through the typical first office visit, from the initial appointment forward. Your first appointment is scheduled following your initial phone call to your orthodontist's office.

1. **On arrival at the office, you will be greeted by one of our certified smile advocates.** She or he is fully prepared to make everything from the first appointment to an entire treatment program go smoothly for you and your child. Your smile advocate will manage your relationship with us, from appointment scheduling for your convenience to answering questions.

At the initial visit, your smile advocate will review your child's patient information and health history and/or any appearance concerns with you.

2. **Next, your orthodontist will conduct the "Customized Smile Analysis,"** the most complete and thorough orthodontic exam, including teeth, gums, mouth, jaws, and face. Typically, safe digital x-rays are taken of the teeth and surrounding bone and of the jaw structures. 3-D Digital scans of the teeth may be made.

Usually that same day, your orthodontist will present his or her "report of findings"—a "show-n-tell," in plain English (not medical jargon), of the full state of your child's teeth, gums, mouth and jaws, and a diagnosis of any present or anticipated problems that should get orthodontic treatment. If treatment should occur, your orthodontist will present recommendations and options. This will be an individualized, personalized plan of treatment, not "braces in a box, off the shelf." By this report of findings, you will know:

- what teeth or jaw misalignment or other problems exist or are developing

- what the health and appearance ramifications are of not intervening with treatment

- if orthodontic therapy is needed now or later and which type of appliances will be best in your situation

- what the complete treatment program will consist of: things like the type of appliance, number of appointments, and average time of each office visit

- what results will be achieved at the end of treatment

3. All your questions will be answered. There are no dumb or embarrassing questions. Every single one of my patients has a question, simple or complex! We do *not* want you or your son or daughter just nodding, then later wondering, "What did he mean by *that?*" or saying, "I wish I'd asked about ..." This is *not* one of those "I'm the doctor—trust me—just do what I say because I said so" offices. Most questions will have been answered by literature provided to you, this book, and your orthodontist's report of findings, but it's a lot to take in. So, any and all questions you have should be asked and answered. Our goal is not just a terrific orthodontic outcome ensuring a healthy, attractive smile, but also your anxiety-free comfort from start to finish.

4. Finally, your smile advocate will explain the costs of the prescribed treatment program and discuss payment arrangements as needed. Before proceeding, the next two appointments will be scheduled for the installation of aligners or braces and/or other treatment. As the saying goes, a journey of a thousand steps begins with the first one, and a task well begun is sooner done!

In total, you should allow about one hour for this entire initial consultation and exam.

If that seems like a lot, keep in mind there are *lifetime* health, appearance, and personality aspects of this. And it's not "installing tires"—not if it's done properly and expertly. Your son or daughter deserves a careful, thorough, and anxieties-eliminated experience. You want to make the best decisions for them.

Frankly, our practice and our process is not for everybody. We attract and "resonate with" parents who are quite serious about their responsibilities and committed to giving their child every possible advantage in life—certainly not unnecessary disadvantages. If you are that parent—and the fact that you took the trouble to obtain and read this book suggests it—then you are going to recognize that this is time well invested in the best possible results.

"Our experience with the orthodontist has been better than we ever expected. My son is so proud of his smile, more and more every day."

—MARY C.

Chapter Six

Shouldn't There Be a Guarantee?

GUARANTEES ARE CONTROVERSIAL IN all kinds of health care, including orthodontics. Many doctors are upset by the very idea. One huffed and puffed at me, "What do you think you're doing with this guarantee nonsense? We aren't operating a car shop, installing mufflers and guaranteeing them for five thousand miles. We are doctors!"

His ego was mightily offended. But I doubt you will be, with the challenge of deciding who should be your family's *trusted* orthodontist. So, yes, I think there should be a guarantee! In fact, many guarantees!

1. **If you aren't satisfied with your son or daughter's orthodontic treatment, new smile outcome, or patient/ parent experience,** *our team of specialists will make it right, guaranteed.*

2. **You also have a safety in numbers guarantee.** The diagnostic and prescriptive methods and state-of-the-art technology and the products we use have been used by top orthodontists nationwide to treat over one million patients successfully.

3. **You also have my guarantee that *every* team member at my office has been not only academically educated but also *thoroughly* trained.** They all follow the same proven method to diagnose needs, plan the best and personalized treatments for every patient, and manage for best results from day one through after-care. All patient care is supervised and reviewed by me. We also invest in frequent state-of-art clinical continuing education for our team.

4. You also have *my guarantee of exceptional courtesy and customer service.* Yes, you are my patient, but we can be honest about this—my practice is not just a health care provider, it is also a *business.* As such, it has, in my opinion, one set of responsibilities to you as the parent of a patient and one set to the patient, including telling the whole truth and nothing but the truth, prescribing in the patient's best interest, and delivering the best possible treatment and outcomes. There's also a second, separate set of responsibilities to you as a customer, including access, convenience, responsiveness, and "red carpet service."

These guarantees are included in your treatment program fee.

For starters, I can guarantee you the best, most thorough orthodontic exam, and I encourage coming in for it now.

Chapter Seven

How to Get More Information

SO, FIRST, THE best thing to do is make certain you get all your questions answered by the orthodontist and the practice's advocate. Don't hold back. Be assertive. Don't feel you have to be deferential to the doctor! My own goal in this is to have every patient and every patient's parent *fully* knowledgeable about every aspect of the treatment so that they have *zero* anxiety.

Second, visit ExcellenceInOrthodontics.org, cao-aco.org, or aaoinfo.org. These are professional organizations who provide carefully curated, vetted, authoritative, accurate, and understandable patient and parent information. These can definitely help you decide on the questions you want answers to.

Finally, ask around. I'd suspect there are a few of your friends, colleagues, and acquaintances who have a friend or family member in orthodontic treatment at our office. Drill them with questions on their experiences, thoughts and feelings about our office.

Now that we know where to get your most burning orthodontic questions answered, here are some simple tips I've amassed over the years to help you easily and effectively get the information you need:

How to Get Your Questions Answered

Make a list. The easiest way to get what you want is to know it in advance. Make a list of the various questions you have when they arise so you can quickly and easily go down the list to assure you've got the right answers for the right questions.

Bring it with you. Take the list with you when you go for your child's orthodontist visit. This way you have the questions at hand at the right place at the right time. If you're calling in to get answers, you can also have the list ready and tick off one question for every answer you receive.

Record the answers. If your orthodontist, or their reception-tionist, speaks too fast or you can't keep up while writing the answers down, why not record them? Your cell phone likely has a "record" feature or we can find a solution such as Go To Meeting.

Double-check. Finally, make sure you have the right answer by double-checking with your orthodontist or one of their team members.

Knowing where to find the information you need is only half the battle; follow these tips and you'll know how to get what you're looking for as well.

Regardless of how many questions you have, or your comfort level with technology, phone calls, or in-person visits, your orthodontist should offer an option that fits your schedule and makes all your unresolved issues crystal clear.

Chapter Eight

How to Pay For Orthodontic Treatment

YOU MAY HAVE NEVER needed braces. Or you may have needed them and gotten them. Or you may be among the tens of thousands of people in our generation who needed them but did not get them, perhaps because your family decided they couldn't afford them. Maybe they didn't consider it a priority and probably underestimated the lifelong results of the decision. You may not only have lived with a "hide your smile" habit unnecessarily, but you may have developed chronic jaw pain and headaches, difficulty chewing, or even periodontal disease that could have been prevented.

Regardless of which group you're in, I hope you will be making the best choices for your child or daughter today, without being hamstrung just by the finances. Truth is, parents pay out the same cost for a number of different things not nearly as vital as health or emotional well-being without blinking, mostly because it's paid in installments or just never really *considered*, like the monthly cost for minutes/data on mobile devices, added up for a year or two. The additional insurance cost and other costs when the teenager gets his driver's permit; after all, what's the choice? The cost of orthodontics leaps up and stands there, all at one time. So, it can seem big. And it tempts thoughts of, "maybe later," or, "is this really necessary?"

I hope in the prior chapters I have succeeded at getting the "is it really necessary?" question erased. If there is visible need or if expert examination by an orthodontist and his explanation of what he finds can show you say it is advisable, it *is* necessary! It won't fix itself. It will probably get worse. It plagues a person's health, emotional well-being, social life, and career. It can link to very serious medical problems. *Necessary* is not really debatable.

Now let's tackle the ugly matter of the money.

I say "ugly" because nobody really likes talking about this. Most orthodontists are nervous about it. Parents are uncomfortable with it. If there is a financial obstacle to treatment, most people are reluctant to admit it, offer other excuses, and then can't be helped by the doctor. I think we have to trust each other. With me, this discussion is entirely confidential, in a "safe zone."

What Is a Reasonable Fee and Cost?

A complete treatment program, including braces, can cost anywhere from $3,500 to $9,500 or so. Most fall in between. Adjusted for inflation, these prices are actually *less than* braces decades ago, while the technology and quality has advanced. In costs it can prevent later, it's a bona fide bargain. TMJ treatments are expensive. Cosmetic dentistry work is expensive. Migraine headache drugs are expensive and have side effects.

For this investment, you will be getting the carefully selected, personalized solution to your child's irregularities and problems, prescribed using state-of-the-art digital technology along with the expertise of a specialist, and considerate, compassionate care from start to finish. Your investment includes a varying number of appointments plus the orthodontic appliance itself, after-care, and in my office, certain guarantees.

It's hard to really draw a fair comparison, but if you have any significant net worth, you can easily pay similar fees for the services of an attorney expert in estate planning. Most kitchen remodels cost considerably more. Where real expertise is involved and the stakes of getting it wrong are high, you can't escape professional level fees.

In this case, the $3,500 to $9,500 range is seen as perfectly reasonable by the overwhelming majority of parents that I talk to. Each year, we provide braces of one kind or another to countless patients. Even parents who shook their heads at the cost to start with tell me afterward that having witnessed everything we do to get the absolute best obtainable results, and seeing the outcome itself, they feel great value.

While it's never easy to part with such a sum, people do it every day for all sorts of less important things, like their new designer handbag, golf vacation, or suite of living room furniture. They'll pay for it outright or with their favorite credit card (getting the reward points in the bargain). If you put the orthodontic treatment program including braces on a typical credit card at the interest in play as I write this, and you choose to make only the minimum required monthly payment, your monthly payments will be relatively small. Even tight budgets can accommodate this *when it is really important.* It's less than most families pay for their cable and streaming entertainment. For many, if they got all their Starbucks stops consolidated into one monthly bill, it would be more than this!

Insurance

These days, there are as many different types of insurance plans as there are patients in my office. I can't possibly speak to your unique and personal insurance policy without seeing it first but, in general, my experience tells me that "most" insurance policies cover "some" of your orthodontic expenses.

I realize that answer sounds very vague, but here are a couple of variables you need to answer before an insurance agent can help you determine what, how long, and how many procedures fall under your insurance:

- the duration of the procedure (two months, six months, a year, etc.)

- the cause of the procedure (a patient presenting with pain, a parent's concern, traumatic injury or accident, congenital birth defect like cleft lip or palate, etc.)

- the nature of the procedure (to correct the bite, pain/ discomfort, cosmetic, etc.)

I can only partially answer this question, but talking to your insurance agent will help you get the right answers you need.

Chapter Nine

What Are the Treatment Options?

IF YOUR CHILD is ready for orthodontic care, one of the first discussions to have with your orthodontist is which procedure is right for him or her; there might be more options than you had ever imagined.

If you're like most people, you associate orthodontists with braces, but these days, that is just one arm of what I or any orthodontist does. Here are some of the services most orthodontists will provide their patients with during the course of routine treatment:

- metal, tie-free braces

- Invisalign clear removable aligners

- clear braces

- expanders to match jaw size and tooth size

- habit appliances to eliminate thumb sucking

- space maintainers

- retainers to prevent crowding and shifting of teeth

- headgear to help correct jaw alignment

- functional appliances to help improve facial balance

- early treatment and growth modification

- customized appliances designed uniquely for each patient

While many of these services may seem self-explanatory to you, several will probably not. In the following pages, I will try to elaborate on several of them, including:

- crossbite correction

- metal braces

- clear braces

- Invisalign

Crossbite Correction

As your child's teeth begin to grow in, there's a *lot* more at work than mere gum lines, tooth fairies, and molar size. How the jaw is shaped, when it develops, and even how "normally" it develops can all affect the placement and comfort of your child's teeth.

When the upper and lower teeth grow at different rates, or even when the lower jaw grows disproportionately with the upper jaw, something known as a "crossbite" can occur.

Your child might have a crossbite if, for instance, the lower jaw is out of line with the upper jaw (kind of like a box that won't close right because one of the hinges is bent).

Or perhaps on the right side of your child's mouth, the lower teeth "stick out" a little farther than the top teeth, making the upper teeth on that side overlap in turn.

Or maybe your child's upper and lower jaws are out of alignment so instead of the top and bottom front teeth meeting "naturally" as they should, the front teeth fall somewhat behind the lower teeth. This would be the reverse of an overbite.

As you might imagine, any or all of these developments can lead to short- and long-term discomfort for your child.

How, When, and Why Crossbites Form

You might be amazed to find out how many ways a crossbite can form as your child grows and develops during his or her formative years. Heredity is one key to jaw growth, or alignment, as is the size of your child's developing jaw.

Another factor that can contribute to the development of a potential crossbite is if it takes your child too long to lose his or her baby teeth. In some extreme cases, in fact, if it takes too long for your child to lose his baby teeth, another set of teeth can grow in behind them, throwing the alignment off and contributing to a crossbite.

Believe it or not, something as basic as whether your child breathes through her nose or her mouth can also contribute to a crossbite. While most children breathe through their noses, some children develop a habit early on of breathing through their mouths instead.

In children who breathe through their noses while they're sleeping, the tongue naturally rests on the roof of the mouth, promoting natural and proper upper jaw growth. When young children breathe through their mouths, however, the tongue relocates from the roof of the mouth to the bottom, removing that extra support and potentially contributing to reduced upper jaw bone growth; this can create the crossbite we spoke of previously.

How Can I Spot a Crossbite?

Although it sounds severe, and even painful from the description provided earlier, the effects of a crossbite can take time to manifest themselves. Still, here are some of the telltale signs your child might be cultivating, or already suffering from, a crossbite:

- snoring

- difficulty breathing

- chewing on one side of the mouth or the other

- signs of an underbite

- if your child's chin seems "off center" or disproportionate

How, When, and Why to Correct a Crossbite

Where should you start looking for treatment if you're concerned about your child's jaw development after reading this section? If you suspect your child might have a crossbite, approach your family dentist about a recommendation for a specialist such as an orthodontist.

There are many possible treatments available for a crossbite, and your orthodontist can work with you closely to make the right and specific decisions for you and your child.

When should you start? I believe you know my standard answer when it comes to questions like this one: *as early as possible*! The same way an auto mechanic would tell you to take care of that oil leak, bulging tire, or faulty timing belt sooner rather than later, myself and my colleagues in orthodontics will always favor early treatment to later.

Crossbites are often closely linked with other orthodontic issues, such as teeth alignment, jaw size, and growth, so naturally, the sooner you address any or all of these issues, the better.

Finally, why should you address a crossbite? Crossbites can lead to pain, discomfort, and a lack of confidence as your child begins to feel insecure or even ostracized because of this very treatable, very normal series of jaw and teeth developments.

Not only can crossbites become physically uncomfortable if left untreated, but if the misalignment or root cause of the bite isn't fixed early in childhood, then the child's appearance and, ultimately, confidence could be affected as the crossbite becomes more pronounced in adolescence.

Metal Braces or Clear Braces

The fact is, braces still have a valued place in the orthodontic world, and despite advances and breakthroughs of products like Invisalign, they aren't going extinct anytime soon! This is because braces are very strong and can withstand most types of treatment. Today's braces are smaller, sleeker, and more polished than ever before.

"Our son has a lot of anxiety about visiting any doctor, but the transition into the orthodontics world was very easy and painless for our family. Thank you for all that you do to bring beautiful smiles to our family and many, many more!"

—MOLLY H.

Older, traditional metal braces require an elastic o-shaped rubber band, called a ligature, to hold the arch wire onto the bracket. These elastic ties collect more plaque and bacteria, making it harder for patients to clean the teeth and gums.

You may have heard of "speed braces." These are sometimes also referred to as "self-ligating brackets" or "tie-free braces." Self-ligating means that the brackets do not need the little o-shaped rubber bands (ligatures) or metal tie wires to hold the arch wire onto the bracket. Several companies have developed braces for holding the wires in place without ligatures.

By using self-ligation technology, the brackets allow the wire to slide back and forth. This advancement allows for fewer adjustments and fewer appointments. These types of braces do not need rubber bands to hold the arch wire in place. They use a "door" to secure the arch wire to the bracket. They're smaller than traditional metal and less food gets trapped around them when you eat.

Orthodontists might use an advanced self-ligating bracket that does not require physical tightening of the wire to the braces. It's a twin bracket made of metal or clear ceramic and utilizes a special built-in clip. The pressure from specific types of arch wires activates the clip and delivers specific amounts of force to each tooth, resulting in fast, directed results.

Naturally, orthodontists are very excited about the hygiene benefits of these self-closing or tie-free metal braces. Patients are excited that their braces are small, smooth, and friction-free, and will straighten their teeth in fewer visits with less discomfort than braces with wires that are "tied-in."

Invisalign

Invisalign is a widely advertised, well-known, and popular braces-alternative, and kids often know about it and ask parents and doctors for it by name. For many, it's as good an option as any other and sometimes even the best option.

Invisalign uses advanced, proprietary 3-D computer-imaging technology which allows your orthodontist to "map" the entire span of treatment, from the present teeth alignment to the desired positioning, alignment, and smile. Clear aligners are custom made and based on the 3-D imaging. Invisalign has many features that have helped make it such a popular choice. The aligners are removable before a snack or meal as well as for general hygiene. There are no metal brackets or wires. Office visits for adjustments throughout the treatment program are fast, easy and painless. The thermoplastic aligners are virtually invisible. Over four million patients have been treated with Invisalign, and there is a special Invisalign system for teens and children.

Because Invisalign is computer mapped, there's sometimes the idea that anybody can install Invisalign and that all practitioners using Invisalign are the same. I have an important warning about this: during each stage of the complete treatment, only certain teeth are allowed to move. Which teeth move in what order, and the amount of time (days/weeks) needed for each successive set of aligners differs for each patient. *This* is what you rely on an expert orthodontist specialist to decide. At the start, we determine whether your son or daughter is a good candidate for the Invisalign approach. As a top level Invsalign provider, and having been mentored by some of the top orthodontists in the field, I feel confident in prescribing Invisalign in most cases. Invisalign technology continues to improve, and I am impressed with the results that I can achieve using this tool. With Invisalign, I can achieve great results—in less time and with cleaner teeth than with traditional braces.

A word of caution—check on the Invisalign website for a top level provider in your area. Invisalign is a tool, so be sure that you have an expert, experienced orthodontist to use it!

Adult Orthodontics

It's not uncommon for individuals who have undergone orthodontic treatment earlier in life to find their teeth have drifted out of alignment over the years. Most adults won't think twice about bleaching their teeth to roll back the effects of time. Yet few think about the role orthodontics can play.

Adults of all ages can enjoy the same cosmetic and health benefits of properly aligned teeth with appliances like Invisalign. Improperly aligned teeth can do more than undermine your confidence. They can make proper cleaning and brushing more difficult, contribute to enamel loss and even set the stage for more significant problems down the road. Fortunately, discrete treatment with aligners or clear braces can help keep you aligned with a healthy, happy lifestyle.

Trustworthy, Objective Advice

Our office is *not* "in the pocket of" or obligated to any of these providers of different braces products and technologies. We select and recommend what we believe is *the* most appropriate and beneficial choice for your child. We are happy to discuss the pros and cons of each, if your child has their heart set on, say, Invisalign, because that's what a friend has, or based on information you've obtained.

The number-one rule here is: what is absolutely best for the patient?

Chapter Ten

Invisalign Teen: Changing Orthodontics for the Better

AS A PRACTITIONER, I like to be on the cutting edge of new technology, because I'm excited about the advantages it can offer my patients. The kinds of digital tools we're using now allow us to customize treatment so effectively that the procedures are significantly shorter in time—that's good news for patients.

Traditionally in orthodontics, patients were looking at about two years of treatment time. Today, with the use of digital technology, we can get people's treatment time down to a year, and sometimes even shorter. I've tried almost everything because I know my patients' time is valuable, and the system I'm most excited about is Invisalign, because of the great results it creates and the speed at which it accomplishes them.

This fully customized treatment is first planned by me on the computer. This allows us to design efficiencies into the treatment, and we can move people to their final result a lot more quickly. The

Invisalign aligners are much easier to live with than old-fashioned braces because they're removable for cleaning and when you eat. I look at it as the modern way to do orthodontics versus the classic braces. A lot of orthodontists dabble in Invisalign, but I've worked to make myself an expert in it and am delighted with the results we get.

Teenagers love Invisalign for all the reasons I've mentioned and also because they're virtually invisible when worn. Probably about half of the younger teens I've treated were fine with the idea of old-fashioned braces, but not the teens who were a little older. Kids from the tenth grade and up didn't want to be identified as "brace face"; they wanted to be seen as adults. One way around that was to put clear braces on our teenage patients so they were less noticeable. But that didn't solve all their problems; some of them had heard from their friends that had been in braces that it's uncomfortable. The rubbing and the discomfort are two other things they struggle with, especially if they're either playing certain sports or musical instruments. If you happen to get an elbow to the cheek or lip while playing basketball—and you're not wearing a mouth guard because it's supposed to be a non-contact sport—the inside of your mouth can get cut up pretty bad.

Eating is another big problem for teens and kids with braces, because so many foods they like are on the "do not eat" list. You can eat hard and sticky foods with aligners—as they're removable—but not with braces, and a lot of kids resent that. They can't eat popcorn, or hard or chewy candies, or chew gum. With braces, kids often ignore or forget the rules, so they break their wires on things like candy apples (or even regular apples) and have to come in for repairs. This is even more of a hassle for the parent tasked with getting them into the office and putting that time aside in their already busy schedule. With Invisalign, that's not an issue, and that's appealing to both parents and teens. While you can't chew gum while wearing aligners, you can otherwise carry on as normal because you take them out when you eat.

Usually, the worst thing that happens—in terms of negative outcomes with braces—is tied to the fact that teens tend to struggle with hygiene and diet throughout their treatment; braces, as you can imagine, can collect a lot of stuff if they're not properly cleaned. This can lead to white spots all over the teeth, called lesions, when we take the braces off. These blemishes are where acid formed from the plaque deposits, creating a weak spot on the enamel, and are a consequence of that poor oral hygiene. In fairness, it's tough keeping teeth clean with braces on; flossing is mandatory, but it's very challenging to floss when you have wires connecting all your teeth. You have to thread it through and practically do needlework to get the floss where it needs to go. Too many kids give up on it and are consequently left with these unwanted spots of decalcification.

When you make the investment to put your teen in braces, you are counting on them to take on new, additional responsibility for their hygiene—in my experience, many kids just won't follow through. I had a mom come in to see me recently; we had a conference because her daughter was struggling with her oral hygiene. The mom was frustrated because it was creating stress and arguments. Raising a teenager is stressful enough, and as parents we've already got plenty of challenges. Kids are struggling with a lot of different things, too, and they're apt to be resistant to their parents. I don't know if you've tried to help your teenager brush his or her teeth lately, but I can tell you most of them won't welcome your help. That was certainly the case with this lady and her daughter; she'd done all she could to encourage, assist, and remind her daughter what her responsibilities were, but it just wasn't working.

After we talked, the mom went home and they talked it out; ultimately, she brought her daughter back to us to remove her braces, and told us, "We're done. I told her we're done."

We said, "Okay, we agree. Let's see what we can do to stabilize what she has and we can revisit this again." Currently, we plan her next move will be to aligners. With aligners, you still have some struggles, but the hygiene issue is much more manageable.

Five years ago, I'd have been pushing this patient away from Invisalign and towards keeping those braces, but improvements in Invisalign technology—and the extensive continuing education we train in to use them most effectively—means that I can accomplish much more with them than in the past.

The biggest challenge with our teenage patients is compliance: keeping them engaged in treatment and coaching them through it. The coaches in our practice are trained to motivate patients and keep them motivated, because if the patient doesn't manage their aligners properly, they're not going to do any good. But as the treatment times are shorter and shorter, the patient is more likely to maintain their routines and follow the program, so we're seeing improved compliance.

It Matters Who Your Doctor Is

Invisalign isn't "plug and play," though there *are* those who would have you believe that anyone can do it. As a practitioner, you actually need to know quite a lot to get the most out of it.

Some orthodontists (and even some general dentists) will take a weekend course or two, and on the basis of that knowledge will set themselves up with the Invisalign system and take on patients. Some of them are treating three or four cases a year. On the other hand, highly experienced practitioners, like my practice, have been treating three or four hundred cases every year. Why would you trust someone with your family's orthodontic care if they are only partially trained? And education has to be ongoing, because the product continues to improve. I'm always taking more courses to stay on top of innovations; I completed a year-long Invisalign master's course on treatment and planning, led by some of the top practitioners in the field, which was transformational for me in terms of tapping the potential of this technology.

The dedication to staying on top of technological advancements pays dividends for my patients. Recently I worked with a patient who'd been told by other orthodontists that the only way to treat her would be through surgery to correct her bite, combined with braces. Five years ago, I would have probably recommended the same thing, and of course, there are still cases in which surgery is the best way to correct real jaw discrepancies—but unsurprisingly, most patients don't want jaw surgery. One of the great things about Invisalign is that we now can use it to close down peoples' open bites and get them fully corrected, without surgery.

I looked at this lady's case and saw that with aligners, I'd be able to move the teeth predictably, control the bite, and compensate for the jaw discrepancy that she has. I told her, "Let's give it a go with the aligners. I believe we can get you there. If we can't, then we always can sit down, regroup, and work out plan B, which would be braces and surgery. Even in that case, the braces will be on for a shorter time than they would have needed to be in the past." To put it mildly, she was relieved to learn she might not need surgery, and her treatment today is still going beautifully.

Teenagers are understandably scared of the word "surgery" and so are their parents, who tend to be very hesitant to make that choice for their kids. It's great to be the guy who has a non-surgical solution for them.

Another advantage of aligners is that they require far fewer office visits than braces do. The average number of visits for a braces patient is twenty; the average for an Invisalign patient is ten, although we're getting it down to six or eight visits. That's less than half the commitment, so there's significantly less impact on your life compared to braces—a large consideration given how busy our kids and we are.

Advances in Invisalign

Thanks to improvements in Invisalign's materials over the last four or five years, we can accomplish so much more than used to be the case. In some especially challenging cases, we're able to come up with a hybrid approach, so we can use braces for the difficult parts that aligners can't do: for instance, an impacted tooth on the patient's palate. As Invisalign continues to modify and improve its system, though, we're moving away from braces at a faster rate.

Three big factors drives Invisalign up to the next level in terms of what it can do. First, the company has invested a lot in research and development (R&D), and has invented its own patented polymer, one that allows aligners to move teeth more efficiently. Second, they hired one of the leading researchers in tooth movement from the University of Connecticut to run the R&D division and improve on the ways in which plastic moves teeth. Under his direction, they have devised a system to put little handles on the teeth called attachments. They're made in different shapes and are engineered to move the teeth very specifically with precise movements. The third thing that's allowed them (and us) to use the product more effectively is all the data they've collected from all the orthodontists that have been working with it. In turn, the data has been used to set up advanced training and mentoring programs. This commitment to continuing innovation means that even people who might have been told they weren't good candidates for aligners in the past can be treated successfully with them now.

Within Invisalign's tiered system of authority and expertise, I am at the "Diamond" level, which is the top 1 percent, and we are the top provider of Invisalign on Vancouver Island. I'm also the top Invisalign Teen Provider. Part of the reason for that is the numbers of teens I treat every year. The other reason is that we've made a real effort to help these patients succeed with the system, and our young patients and their parents are delighted with their results.

Smile Faster with Treatment Accelerators

We're getting help from technology in other ways, too, including devices designed to make teeth move more quickly. Treatment accelerators are housed in a little wafer that the patient bites down on. They use it for five minutes of the day, every day at home. We find it's best if the patient sets aside a specific time to use it every day.

What the treatment accelerator does is to stimulate blood flow and thus the cells in the bone that need to adapt and turn over the bone as we move teeth through the bone. It allows the teeth to move more freely, faster and more comfortably. In fact, we've found we can move teeth from 30 percent to 50 percent faster in those patients who faithfully use it as directed—but again, compliance can be an issue, especially with teens. Fortunately, teens' teeth move pretty quickly already, and the adults who do need it more tend to be better at remembering to use it.

As you can see, most of this technology is designed to shave off weeks and months from the treatment phase of orthodontics, and for a good reason. People hate that second year of treatment. The first year, they can see the dramatic changes, but by the second year, the pace of change slows down and is less evident. The kids especially just think we're punishing them. They finally get to celebrate when they get their braces off and at that point, they like us again, but there's a period of time in the middle where even the nicest patients turn grumpy and all they can focus on is "I want to get these off because they're such a hassle."

Invisalign eliminates so much of that hassle that it's rapidly becoming the treatment of choice for adults and teens. Even if you've been told in the past that you weren't a good candidate for aligners, or if you or your teen have put off getting needed orthodontic treatment because you didn't want the discomfort and hassle of braces, now's the time to get a new opinion. The advances I talked about above make it much more likely that your case can be successfully treated with Invisalign, and we're dedicated to finding a way to make it work for you.

If we have recommended Invisalign and it turns out not to be a good fit, as long as dental hygiene is a good, we can easily switch to traditional braces for no extra charge.

Chapter Eleven

How Difficult Is Living with Braces

REMEMBER, THIS ISN'T 1982. Or 1992. Today's braces aren't anything like yours if you had them decades ago. Today's orthodontic care is far more advanced, more sophisticated, and more patient-centered than any prior generation has experienced. If you had traditional metal braces twenty years or so ago, you experienced medieval torture. The dungeon is gone too, replaced by ultra-modern, comfortable, and patient-friendly offices. Out of the dark, into the light!

Living with today's orthodontic appliances are *not* going to be anywhere near as difficult as you might imagine.

Let's look at a few specific concerns.

Brushing and Hygiene

Modern braces, whether they're metal, flexible, or "invisible," are all actually made to fit the individual and facilitate easy, painless, thorough brushing. This means your child brushes pretty much the same as he would if he didn't have braces.

Here are some simple tips you can share with your child for the best results when brushing with braces on:

- Brush your teeth with a soft or extra-soft nylon toothbrush after you eat and before bed.[2]

- Brush, rinse, and look; if you find any areas that are not clean, brush them again.

- Brush your gums as you brush your teeth (massage and stimulate).

- Take extra care in the area between the gums and the braces because food caught and left there can cause swollen gums, cavities, discomfort, and permanent teeth stains.

- Floss your teeth at least once daily.

- If no toothpaste is available, brush without.

- If you are unable to brush, rinse your mouth vigorously with water.

- Replace your old toothbrush when it gets worn out.[3]

---

2   At my office, you'll be provided with a home kit which will help you take care of your teeth and gums during treatment.

3   You should be replacing your toothbrush every three months regardless, and immediately after you have been ill (as harmful bacteria can remain on your brush).

- It's absolutely essential you continue regular visits to your family dentist for checkups and cleanings throughout your orthodontic treatment!

Depending on the age of your child, you, the parent, may need to supervise the first few brushings.

Forbidden Foods Your Child Must Avoid

After your child's orthodontic appliances have been placed, the teeth are usually "tender" and sensitive for as few as three to as many as ten days: a *short* time. During these few days, softer foods are recommended: soups, macaroni, spaghetti, eggs, fish, Jell-O, yogurt. As needed, Tylenol or Advil are adequate in relieving any discomfort, taken an hour or so before eating. Warm saltwater rinses can be helpful. We also provide a "soft white wax," a safe topical that eases gum discomfort.

For the entire duration of the braces being in place, I'd advise you to stay away from hard and sticky foods that can damage braces and may lengthen the time they have to be worn or even require extra office visits. Sugar-rich foods can make hygiene harder and cause calculus build-up and cavities. You're probably already monitoring and limiting your child's intake of such foods, so there's really nothing new under the sun here. But, for the record, here are the "featured items" that should be avoided during orthodontic treatment and wearing of braces:

1. **Hard foods**: ice (don't chew ice!), nuts, popcorn (has hard kernels inside), peanut brittle, rock candy, whole apples and carrots (unless cut into bite sized pieces), corn on the cob, hard pretzels, hard rolls, hard taco shells.

2. **Extra-sticky foods**: Jolly Ranchers or Starbursts or similar candies, bubble gum, taffy, and sticky cinnamon rolls.

3. **Very chewy foods**: pizza crust, beef jerky, gummy bears. Note: no chewing on pencils or pens.

4. **Super sugary foods and drinks**: soda pop with sugar, ice cream, most cookies, and cake. Yes, this is the worst of the forbidden foods. Some kids will give you a tough time. But there are sugar-free versions of all these kinds of foods, to be made, baked, or store-bought.

We will speak about this with your son or daughter and give them a printed list, but *you* will have to reinforce, monitor, and provide some substitute foods to prevent mutiny or months of sulking. Most kids get it, though. When they understand how short or long the number of weeks of wearing orthodontic appliances will turn out to be, how comfortable or uncomfortable wearing them is, how maintaining hygiene while wearing them is, and how their results are linked to them staying away from the short list of harmful foods, they are pretty responsible about it. Most parents who are initially really worried about this tell us later it wasn't the horror show they'd imagined.

Emergencies, Injuries, Travel, and Time Away from Home

Many "emergencies" actually aren't and can be easily and safely remedied at home. Common emergencies include the breaking of some part of the braces. These sort of things are addressed in the "What to Do" instructions.

If you do run up against an emergency that isn't easily managed with these instructions or if you can't wait for regular office hours, we have a special phone number to call that routes to a knowledgeable staff member directly and who will return your call within sixty minutes or less.

If your family or son or daughter are away from home and, say, they chomp down on a piece of toffee and break a piece of their braces, there is *always* a remedy. You are *not* going to cut your vacation short and rush to the airport! Again, often a remedy provided by our instructions can meet the urgent need until everybody gets back home.

Here is just how good the appliances themselves and our management of orthodontic treatment has gotten. In 2016 to 2017:

- Ninety-eight percent of patients required *no* extra office visits for repairs, adjustments, care, or emergencies beyond their regularly scheduled office visits per their treatment plan.

- Eighty-five percent of patients called with questions, worries, or emergencies that were handled simply by advice and home remedy and/or waited without harm until the next regularly scheduled visit.

- Only 2 percent of patients had some problem or emergency requiring an extra, unscheduled office visit.

Sports

Speaking of injuries, the question of sports versus braces worries kids and parents alike. These days, kids are *very* active in organized and school sports, some starting one as another's season is ending. You know this; you are coordinating the schedules and working as their unpaid chauffeur.

Good news: for every sport and every level of play, there is either an inexpensive off-the-shelf mouth guard or a slightly costlier, custom-fit mouth guard to provide an extra, suitable level of dental protection and to protect the braces themselves. In some sports, additional face masks or other equipment normally treated as an option can be added and used during the time period of the orthodontic treatment. Ask us for guidance for your child and their sport(s). Some mouth guards even come with insurance against dental injury, covering financial costs.

We have thought this through! For example, research reported in *Clinics in Sports Medicine*—from the Department of Neurology at Boston University School of Medicine—examined uses of different kinds of mouth guards and the rate of sports-related concussions. There was no significant difference in concussion risks found tied to different types of mouth guards. We can select the best one for your child, their sport, and the level of play and, if a factor, your budget with no worry about one choice instead of another affecting risk of concussion.

This, by the way, is typical of a good orthodontic specialist: attention to *every* detail. They should have a good knowledge of every ramification of wearing orthodontic appliances, clinical and technological advancements, and every patient or parent need. To be blunt, it's a practical impossibility for a general dentist to give the braces work he does on the side anywhere near this same level of all-in focus.

By the way, there are collegiate and pro athletes—even NFL players—getting orthodontic treatment and even wearing braces. If they can, your child can! You do *not* need the drama of stopping your child from playing the sports they're committed to because of their orthodontic treatment.

See, this *isn't* going to be difficult!

Tips for Helping Your Child Adjust to a Life During Orthodontic Treatment

- **All the cool kids are doing it (or soon will be):** Braces are a very popular appliance during the middle school and high school years. Rather than focus on how he or she feels wearing braces, encourage your child to begin actively looking for other kids who are in treatment. Chances are, they'll find lots more than they ever imagined!

- **Even famous people do it:** Gwen Stefani. Prince Harry. Drew Barrymore. Tom Cruise. Dakota Fanning. Danny Glover. The list of famous people who've worn braces—many of them as adults—could fill half this book. Share with your child how even the most famous people in the spotlight sometimes need a little help through braces.

- **Fast forward:** Many orthodontists provide a "before and after" consultant's session, much like a plastic surgeon. Digital pictures are often used to portray what the child's teeth might look like once the teeth have been straightened and the appliances have been removed. Have your child focus on the "after" when he or she gets down about the "before" shots!

- **Be prepared:** Finally, create a "master list" of things your child likes to do, things that make them feel special, confident, brave, calm, relaxed, or excited. If you notice them feeling down, consult your list and make plans to do something special in the near future to boost their confidence level back to where you know it belongs!

Chapter Twelve

Life After Orthodontics: Retainers

SO, YOUR CHILD'S BRACES are off and they're ready to live a life full of confidence and good oral health. They may think, *I'm free! I'm free!* Well, not quite yet.

The selection of the right orthodontic appliance, the expert orthodontist, and the compliant wearing of the appliance gets us about three-quarters of the way to where we want to be: a well-aligned, as-perfect-as-possible, healthy smile for life.

But after orthodontics, there are retainers.

While many patients are understandably eager to be done with braces once they come off, the fact is, retainers do as much work—if not more—than the braces themselves. Straight teeth in proper alignment have to stay that way, and for that, retainers are a big help.

When appliances are removed, teeth can still shift if not helped through a period of adjustment to settle in. Retainers gently but purposefully remind the teeth to stay straight during this adjustment period. It's advised that nearly all patients who've gone through the time, work, and expense of orthodontics will want to use fixed or removable retainers for months or years or even for life and continue to schedule regular orthodontic checkups. Some dentists doing orthodontics won't tell you this, but I will. Years ago, clinicians believed that once teeth were straightened by braces, they would simply stay that way forever. New science says otherwise. In fact, teeth position shifting as we age is to be expected. Teeth naturally shift to the middle and crowd. So, retainers are actually extremely important in maintaining the new smile from braces. Any claims otherwise, by some "brand" of braces or any doctor, are flat-out false.

Retainers can play a role in:

- closing any gaps that may remain in the bite

- correcting any speech problems—sometimes occurring with a new bite or jaw position

- tongue thrust—where the tongue slips under the teeth while talking

- bruxism—grinding teeth while sleeping

As you can see, there's a lot more to this than just "installing and removing appliances."

In post-orthodontic monitoring and checkups, I tend to decide on the best kind of retainer for your child before the removal of the appliances. Growth of the jaw following treatment (yes, the jaw is still growing in adolescents, to age eighteen or so), stabilization of the gums and bone tissues, pressures from lips and tongue, and other factors tell me what type of retainer should be worn and for how long. Retainers are made out of rubber, plastic, and sometimes, still, metal.

They are custom made and fit as part of the complete orthodontic treatment. However, after the initial orthodontic exam, at the same time the best appliances are being selected, it's usually possible, with a good degree of certainty, to predict the type of retainer(s) your child is going to need, and I'm happy to share that information with you at that time.

Some retainers are invisible or nearly invisible. There are clear plastic retainers. A *fixed* retainer is typically placed on the inside/back surfaces of the lower front teeth. A fixed retainer may be used until lower jaw growth is complete and then no longer needed. When your child hears "retainer" he will most likely picture a *removable* retainer. These make hygiene easy, are easily removed and cleaned daily, and can be removed for a sports activity. There are even "fashion retainers" now—popular with kids of different ages—in school colors, and some even with pictures on them! In my office, patients using different kinds of retainers also receive clear, flexible plastic retainers as a back up in case of damage to the main retainer or for occasional social functions where the preteen or teen "just can't be caught dead with a retainer in his or her mouth."

This is an important part of orthodontic aftercare and part of the complete orthodontic treatment program personalized for your child.

Chapter Thirteen

Let's Celebrate!

HAVING TO WEAR BRACES or aligners can last for six months to two years or more in certain cases. During the time your child has them, they may have moved from child to preteen or preteen to teen, at times feeling embarrassed by having them, and possibly missing out on some things. They probably gave up favorite foods and snacks. They at least had to be super-conscious of what they ate and didn't eat. It's been a long time since they could sink their teeth into an apple or eat popcorn at the movies!

You endured whatever complaining there was. You traded time to the office visits. You dealt with the "uh-oh!" and the "now what did you do?" emergencies if there were any. And, of course, you paid the bill.

We like to see our patients celebrate getting their braces off. There are so many ways your child can celebrate, everything from writing a journal about their experience to recording a video that shares their experience and shows their new look.

Here are a few options your child may want to consider:

- **Throw a party.** Throwing a "braces are off" party is a great way to celebrate. They can invite their friends over, put out the foods that they've been longing for, and they can enjoy showing off those new straight teeth. Their friends will love being able to take part in the celebration.

- **Plan a photo shoot.** Your child deserves to show the world their new beautiful smile! Plan a photo shoot, so they can be one-on-one with a photographer and put their best smile forward. They'll get some great shots and can show all their friends on social media their new look.

- **Chew some sugar-free gum.** Your child might have wanted to have gum for the longest time. Although it's not the best habit, they can take an afternoon to chew some gum and feel guilt and worry free. Chew to your heart's content!

- **Go caramel.** Now is the time your child can sink their teeth into something like a caramel apple. No more avoiding the caramel and cutting the apple into bite-sized pieces. Nope, they can actually eat a full caramel apple, right off the stick! They can get one at the mall or a carnival or even make one themselves. Either way, they'll love being able to bite into that sticky gooey sweetness worry free!

- **Picnic in the park.** Weather permitting, a picnic in the park will make for a fun celebration. Take some of your child's favorite outdoor games, invite the friends, and have a cooler filled with icy drinks. On the grill, you can plan for things like corn on the cob that your child had to largely avoid while wearing their braces. It will make for a memorable afternoon!

- **Have a potluck dinner**. Have your child's friends and family each bring a dish people with braces have to take precaution with. This will give them the chance to learn a little more about what you went through, and it'll be fun to see what options they come up with. Ask each of the guests to write down a comment about your child with or without her braces. Your potluck will be filled with interesting dishes, laughs, and a good time!

- **Relax**. What could be better than spending a couple of hours being pampered, or perhaps a round of golf or fishing out on the lake? Not much! Take your child out—celebrate them making it through their treatment. They'll walk out feeling and looking great!

Doing some of these things, such as chewing gum, may still not be good for your child's teeth or their body overall. But doing it on a special occasion, and not making a habit out of it, won't cause any harm.

Of course, nobody can celebrate unless we *started*. There really is no time like the present.

Chapter Fourteen

What About My Smile?

I'M GOING TO BE honest: if orthodontic treatment was advised when you were eight or ten or twelve and, for whatever reason, it didn't happen, and you now have misaligned teeth, periodontal problems because of them, a smile you often hide, and/or jaw/TMJ pain, it may *not* be an easy fix. It may *not* even be fixable with orthodontics. But, often to the surprise of adults, orthodontics can do a significant amount of good for people thirty, forty, or even fifty years old. You may still be able to go from an embarrassing smile you often hide to a beautiful smile you love! You'll also be able to enjoy better oral health, gently and gradually, over six to twelve months without having teeth pulled and without surgery. Many adults see ten years of age disappear from their faces!

The only way to know what the options are is with a complete, expert orthodontic exam. You can arrange for your exam by speaking to any of the smile advocates at the office.

It's important to get your son or daughter the orthodontic care they need at the earliest time they are known to need it and for it to be the best care available. When that doesn't happen, it often comes around to really bite that person later in life!

Start loving your smile!

"After years of being told I needed surgery, my results are amazing without it. I'm finally able to smile in holiday photos."

—MICHAEL R.

FAQ

Here is a handy resource guide of frequently asked questions and orthodontic terminology, many of which are answered throughout the book.

What might happen if your child's mouth doesn't quite "fit"?

The fact is, the sooner you straighten your child's smile, the faster it will develop as it should: straight, clean, and healthy!

Are there any celebrities who've worn braces?

Many! Gwen Stefani, Prince Harry, Drew Barrymore, Tom Cruise, Dakota Fanning, Danny Glover, and more.

Can I see what my child's straight teeth might look like before the procedure is done?

Yes! 3-D Digital pictures are often used to portray what the child's teeth might look like once the braces have been removed.

Will I be able to afford my child's braces?

Not only are most orthodontic procedures cheaper than ever, but insurance, payment plans, and a variety of other financing options make braces more affordable than they've ever been.

Will getting braces be painful for my child?

Not anymore! Modern technology—and choosing the right orthodontist—can ensure that your child enjoys a pain-free orthodontic experience.

How much school will my child miss because of braces?

Not much, actually. After initial visits and, barring the actual procedure itself, most visits and/or adjustments are routine and can take anywhere from fifteen to forty-five minutes.

Is it really such a big deal if my child has crooked teeth?

Unfortunately, yes. Eroding, crooked, or unaligned smiles can take time to happen, but the time to act is now. Orthodontic irregularities don't just heal on their own or "go away" if you ignore them.

What are some of the warning signs that my child might need to go to the orthodontist?

There are many, but here are a few of the most common: early or late loss of teeth, protruding teeth, grinding or clenching of teeth, and speech difficulty.

What kind of "side effects" are caused by crooked teeth?

Some of the more frequent ones I see include headaches, toothaches, mouth breathing, chipped or worn down teeth, snoring, and drooling.

What makes an orthodontist more qualified than a dentist?

Orthodontists are *dental specialists* who have completed two to three years of additional education beyond dental school to learn the proper way to align teeth and jaws.

Why should I choose a specialist for my child's orthodontic care?

Unique treatment requirements and otherwise difficult bite problems are common, everyday scenarios for your orthodontist. In the interest of receiving the most efficient and effective orthodontic treatment possible, choose an orthodontic specialist.

How do I know if my doctor is an orthodontist?

Only orthodontists can belong to the American Association of Orthodontists (AAO). To find out more, go to aaoinfo.org or cao-aco.org.

What is a smile advocate?

During your initial consultation(s), you will usually be assigned a patient contact person—we call this person a "smile advocate" in our office—with whom you will schedule appointments, confer with rescheduling, and of course, answer any and all questions you may have.

Why are follow-up visits important?

These are wonderful opportunities to either a) ask questions you may have missed the first time, or b) get further details from your orthodontist him- or herself.

Why is early treatment so important?

Age seven is the earliest time your orthodontist can determine future jaw and tooth alignment. That's because, at the age of seven, your child's upper and lower permanent front teeth are developing. These teeth set the stage for future jaw position and serious problems can develop if they come into the wrong position.

Is there such a thing as a child being too old for braces?

Actually, there is. Case in point: waiting to take your child to the orthodontist until they are twelve or thirteen can sometimes make treatment more lengthy, complex, and costly.

What if I don't believe in early orthodontics?

Well, you're entitled to your opinion, but this is like saying you don't believe in the sun. You can hide from it, pretend it's not there, or refuse to acknowledge it, but the simple fact remains. If you're not aware of the potential risks, you can get burnt.

Will my child actually need braces at seven?

Probably not. While I inform parents their child needs an initial exam at age seven, I also mention that most children *will not need braces until eleven to thirteen years of age.*

What is a crossbite?

When the upper and lower teeth grow at different rates, or even when the lower jaw grows disproportionately with the upper jaw, something known as a "crossbite" can occur.

Where should I start to look for treatment if I'm concerned about my child's jaw development?

If you suspect your child might have a crossbite or other issues, approach your family dentist and ask about orthodontics.

Why should I address a crossbite?

Crossbites can lead to pain, discomfort, and lack of confidence as your child begins to feel insecure or even ostracized because of this very treatable, very normal series of jaw and teeth developments.

What is Invisalign?

The Invisalign system is the virtually invisible way to straighten your teeth and achieve the dazzling smile you've always dreamed of. Using advanced 3-D computer-imaging technology, Your orthodontist depicts your complete treatment plan, from the initial position of your teeth to the final desired position.

What are the primary benefits of Invisalign?

Like the word that inspired them, Invisalign aligners are practically clear and as close to "invisible" as one can get. No one may even notice you're wearing these virtually invisible braces, making Invisalign a seamless fit with your lifestyle and day-to-day interactions with others. They are more efficient and more comfortable than traditional braces.

How do I get started with Invisalign?

It's simple: just make an appointment with your local orthodontist for an initial consultation. Most doctors will offer a free initial consultation to see if you are a good candidate for Invisalign.

How will Invisalign effectively move my teeth?

Aligners are the foundation for, and work in unison with, the Invisalign system. Like brackets and arch wires are to braces, Invisalign aligners move teeth by using the appropriate placement of controlled force on your child's teeth.

How many patients are being treated with Invisalign?

More than one million patients worldwide have been treated with Invisalign. The number of Invisalign smiles grows daily.

Is Invisalign appropriate for my child?

Yes, especially because Invisalign now has a system designed specifically for teens and children!

How does Invisalign Teen work?

Aligners snap on your teeth easily. They are comfortable and practically invisible. Invisalign Teen allows permanent teeth to grow and gently and continuously moves your teeth in small increments. Aligners are worn for about two weeks, then you swap them for a new pair.

Why are metal braces still so popular?

Metal braces are very strong and can withstand most types of treatment. Today's metal braces are smaller, sleeker, and more polished than ever before.

What if my child has a "braces emergency" before or after office hours?

If you are experiencing an orthodontic emergency that can't wait for regular office hours, most orthodontic offices have a special number to call, either before, during, or after business hours. If this information isn't given to you readily, ask how your doctor's office handles emergencies.

Can a salt water rinse help deal with irritation caused by braces?

Absolutely; warm saltwater rinses soothe the cheek lining, which can get aggravated by your child's braces.

How do I make a salt water rinse?

To make a salt water rinse, mix half a teaspoon of table salt in one cup of warm water. Stir until the salt is completely dissolved. Gently swish about a fourth of the cup in your mouth for thirty seconds. Make sure you force the water over the areas that feel sore. Then spit the water into the sink. Repeat until the entire cup is gone.

What if my child plays sports and needs a mouth guard?

The best advice for patients or parents looking for a mouth guard can be obtained from your pediatrician, dentist, pediatric dentist, orthodontist or oral surgeon. All of these specialists are uniquely trained to offer customized advice in order to help you prevent a sports-related dental or facial injury.

What about brushing with braces?

Here are some simple tips you can share with your child for the best results when brushing with braces on:

- Brush your teeth with a soft or extra-soft nylon toothbrush after you eat and before bed.

- Brush, rinse, and look; if you find any areas that are not clean, brush them again.

- Brush your gums as you brush your teeth (massage and stimulate).

- If no toothpaste is available, brush without.

- If you are unable to brush, rinse your mouth vigorously with water.

- Replace your old toothbrush when it gets worn out.

- It is absolutely essential that you continue regular visits to your family dentist for checkups and cleanings throughout your orthodontic treatment!

What type of foods should my child avoid while wearing braces?

There are four main types of food your child should avoid while wearing braces: (1) **hard foods**, like ice, popcorn, peanut brittle, rock candy, and corn on the cob, (2) **sticky foods**, like caramels, bubble gum, taffy, and suckers, (3) **chewy foods**, like pizza crust, crusty breads, beef jerky, and gummy bears, and (4) **sugary foods and drinks**, like cake, ice cream, cookies, pie, candy, and soda pop.

Why are retainers so important?

As we age, teeth naturally shift to the middle and crowd. Combined with late growth of the lower jaw, shifting of the teeth is expected following orthodontic treatment. Therefore, retainers are extremely important in the maintenance of your new smile following orthodontic treatment.

Resources

Before or after your consultation, you may want more information for yourself or your son or daughter. The following websites provide valuable insight to help you make the right decision for your child.

Braces.org is the "all about braces site" of the American Association of Orthodontists. This is the official regulatory body and professional association of orthodontists, and *only* orthodontists (*not* dentists) can be members. Here you will receive accurate, up-to-date information on orthodontics.

ExcellenceInOrthodontics.org is the elite association of orthodontists subscribing to a pledge of clinical and customer services excellence. A complete collection of information for patients and parents can be found here.

THE
NEXT
STEP

Your Customized Smile Analysis

When you are ready, I urge you to schedule your Customized Smile Analysis, complete with a complimentary consultation, safe, digital x-rays, an exam, and a report provided to you and your son or daughter—all without cost or obligation.

Call us at **844-240-6688** or go to **oeosmiles.com**.

Printed in the USA
CPSIA information can be obtained
at www.ICGtesting.com
JSHW012039140824
68134JS00033B/3146